Anointed with Oil
The Power of Scent

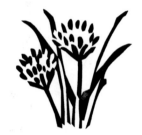

By

Glenda Green
M.A., D.D.

Spiritis Publishing

S

Published by: Spiritis Publishing
P.O. Box 239
Sedona, AZ 86339
www.lovewithoutend.com

Cover design by Alecia Jensen, www.aleciajensen.com

Cover painting: *"Source of Life,"* an original painting by
Glenda Green ©2004.

Printed in the United States of America

ISBN: 0-9666623-5-0

The Sacred Oils mentioned in this book
are available through Spiritis Publishing as well as a growing number of
fine shops.

For more information about them, please visit our website at
www.lovewithoutend.com
Or call our toll free number
1-888-453-6324

To all I have loved, who showed me the ways of life.

Table of Contents

Introduction

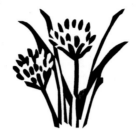

Scent defies the ordinary mind. Though it is one of our five major senses, supplying our brains with a steady stream of environmental information, scent is not a feature of the intellect. It is a powerful experiential force, created to be that way for our very survival. Now we have good reason to believe that it may also facilitate our survival on more than the physical level.

Fragrance and our sense of smell hold a unique place within our consciousness. Smell is our oldest, most primitive sense, in that it is directly received into the primal part of our brain, which directly triggers the autonomic nervous system. This is so that smell can stimulate an immediate survival response without first engaging our cognitive faculty, which might be too slow or wrong. Of all our senses, smell is the most intimately associated with our emotions and feelings, and therefore it is indelibly entwined with our entire emotional response system and history. In many therapeutic healing sessions, practitioners have reported the patient to remember a smell associated with the trauma being addressed, and upon full recognition of the scent, the injury was gone. At the same time, smell is the one sense most reported and associated with miracles or the attainment of higher consciousness. Many who have experienced a miraculous healing have reported a beautiful fragrance, even though no external cause was present.

Could it be that through aroma, we may have a valuable key that unlocks the door to all levels of consciousness, even the hidden ones that hold our forgotten trauma and the higher ones that remind us of the sunlit palaces of Paradise? Indeed, in my experience, aromas present a golden thread that weaves its way through our physical body, while engaging a larger emotional matrix that connects, supports, and directs our physical behavior even beyond that into a larger metaphysical body which serves as a direct link between body and soul. Scent has revealed to me that our body is gradiently linked to our soul, much as material objects represent gradient degrees of compressed or condensed light, ever progressing from the infinite into form…and back again to the infinite. In this, I am assured that our body is just the visible portion **of our soul** and not a separate entity seeking (or avoiding) a spiritual life.

It was within such a state of connection between the infinite and the finite, that I first realized the powerful connection that aroma can provide for uniting the higher dimensions of our being with the physical one on which we all too often fix our attention. There is a holistic nature to scent, whether it is the fragrance of a country garden or the most complex blend of essential oil. Because scent is not refracted by the lens of mental structure, it leads us to an immersed union with experiential moments, and invites us to be anointed by the very essence of our moment in time. Perhaps there is an even greater wholeness to which our sense of smell is attuned…the wholeness of life itself.

Many of you were possibly drawn to this book by your familiarity with my earlier books in which I tell the story of my mystical experience with Jesus Christ. What prompted that unexpected but blessed encounter was a painting of him that I had been inspired to create in 1992. This was a profound experience for me, which united my perception of heaven and earth. One of the more delightful aspects of it is that his presence always brought forth an incomparably beautiful fragrance. Though my studio was saturated with the smell of turpentine and oil paint, I could smell nothing but the extraordinary fragrance that he brought with him every day. It filled my senses, enlivened my being, opened my heart, and illumined my soul. After he left, I could still remember the rare perfume as if it hovered around me.

At the time of that experience I had no familiarity with fragrances other than those provided by nature and, of course, that exceptional one, which had awakened my senses to a higher world. Fortunately, my early life in rural Texas taught me to love the potent smells of the earth and the electrically charged air of weather changes. I was a nature child, as sensitive to smell as the wild baby animals I adopted or the horses I rode. Galloping across the still open rangeland, I could tell where there was water almost as soon as my horse could. In my middle years I was blessed to own a vineyard, and that was an education in the cultivated understanding of aroma. I could smell the bouquet of grapes and know as they matured what kind of harvest it would be. More than that, I began to recognize the holistic nature of what scent revealed. My love of scent is deeply rooted in my personal history, although I never expected to have mystical experiences that would also reveal to me the fragrances of higher realms. As a result of having such a broad range of experience with scent, I now realize that scent may be our most universal sense, from basic survival (smelling danger, safety, water, or food) to the highest experiences of the soul or consciousness.

So, there I was in 1992, presented with a desire and a challenge. I yearned to recreate the most heavenly aroma I had ever encountered. The problem was I knew nothing about the blending aromas. My first move was to contact people who did know something about the subject. My excitement not withstanding, I was unfortunately headed for a nosedive. It did not take me long to realize that it would be pointless to engage the exceptional skill and talent of others, if I did not know the basics of fragrance myself. I could not even describe the aroma I hoped to create, much less use the technical terms which form the everyday language of aromacology. What was a 'top note', a middle note', a base 'note' or a fixative? It all sounded more like music than chemistry.

Thus my education began in 1993. That was followed by experience, intuitive exploration, and creative experimentation. There was also the intimidating reality of markets, sources, and world supply. Much like fine wine, essential oils are only as good as the source plant and the processes by which they are refined. One can add to that the fact that there are "vintage years," ideal climates, and growing fields...preferably wild.

Try though I did, I could not replicate the scent of Christ through a technical approach—even with the help of talented aromacologists. There was something exceptionally holistic about that fragrance, which defied the assemblage of it from isolated ingredients. The "whole" of the fragrance I sought was so much more than the sum of its parts it could not be captured by estimating and predicting the separate ingredients that would combine to make it.

This was my first realization as to why in the Scriptures certain blends were held to be sacred, and why the priests of old were also alchemists and perfumers of the first order. They had the ability to first sense and envision the perfect fragrance as a creation of God and then allow that perfect fragrance to instruct their intuitive consciousness as to the right formula for its making on earth. That perfect fragrance to them was the breath of God.

I realized that I would only be able to replicate the fragrance by restoring within myself the essence of that original miraculous experience, and then expressing it through the discovery of fragrances. So, for the next ten years, I cultivated my memories of that sacred event and transposed them into a new life of teaching, and writing about my *"Conversations With Jesus"* through the experience of painting his portrait. While I was reassembling my own inner consciousness, I continued to study the arts and science of aroma.

Fortunately I was blessed with good teachers, and I learned with depth and sensitivity. Preparation for the eventual revelation was, however, long and complex. My years of devotion to painting and other art forms led me to expect and cultivate the layers of insight and discernment that would be necessary to refine my perceptions and expressions and shape them into subtle and powerful communications. My years on the vineyard gave me insight and experience into the richness of nature's fruits and the mastery necessary to evaluate and combine them into the most wonderful juices and wines. Slowly I grew into my newest expression of art under divine guidance, love, study of plant essences, support from others who respected my devotion, and perhaps a bit of instinctive ability.

I surmised from the beginning that Frankincense and Myrrh would be two of the ingredients in the aroma of Christ's presence. The question, however, was *which* Frankincense and *which* Myrrh. I had more than a hundred samples of each to examine, and no two were alike. In combination, the possibilities were multiplied. There were a number of points where I would have wilted had this not been a true calling for me.

To some degree all great art has that challenge. It begins with an idea or a vision, and then unfolds through complete surrender to intuitive expression, exploration, and creation. Priests and perfumers of old surrendered to their belief that the Creator of life was the formulator and artist for all anointing oils. There is much truth to that, for without the life force, which essential oils convey, the resulting fragrances would only be for adornment and luxury. Without a higher guidance to formulate the blends, they would never arrive at their consummate clarity and beauty.

The driving force was always to recreate the divine fragrance that filled my days, my dreams, and my waking consciousness while Jesus and I were together. That was the simplicity of my goal. After ten years of much learning, trial, and error, I was ready to be filled with the final inspiration, and the formula came into being in the autumn of 2001. That fragrance is what is known today as

'ChristScent'.   Shortly thereafter I receive the spiritual instructions and grace to create more inspired blends, as well as the greater understanding of the spiritual and physical connections that they revealed.

While this book is documented with many scientific facts and practical uses of essential oils, I must say from the beginning that were it not for the mystical revelations in my life I would neither have become a blender of oils nor would I have written this book. I am devoted to what I have perceived as the holistic union that can be facilitated between body and soul through the use of aromatic blends. I also believe this is a universal subject that need not be attached to any particular belief system.   What I have discovered has also been discovered by healers and mystics all over the world, from time immemorial, within and beyond all belief systems.   Therefore, even though some parts of this book are indelible entwined with my divine guidance and the fruits of it, I will endeavor to make this treatment as valuable as possible from a universal perspective, for it does indeed fill a niche left blank by other treatments of essential oils.

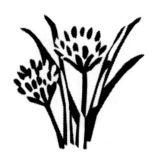

Chapter 1

The Power of Scent

Surely, we all have strolled into the woods, meadows, or a back yard garden at some time to become awash with nature's perfume. It could have been the captivating fragrance of Jasmine or honeysuckle that lured us to follow its path, the fresh smell of grass that gladdened our hearts, or the refreshing aroma of pine, spruce, or juniper that caused us to relax and linger. We are anointed by spirit and life whenever we immerse ourselves in the natural world. In such moments, we are included in nature's vital network of communication, and we are made more whole and more united with all of life. These marvelous refreshing experiences are facilitated by plants as they broadcast their living essential oils. It is their way of communicating among themselves and all the other species of life.

The environment in which man emerged was not only lush but also richly aromatic. Many ancient records give account of man's love of scent. Since the dawn of recorded history, fragrant smoke and other scents have been used in daily rituals and religious ceremonies as a devotion to the all-pervasive Power of life and creation. Fragrance has been referred to as the presence of God on earth, a delicate and precious emanation revealing the connection between spirit and matter. The Bible, from its earliest chapters to the end, is full of references to herbs, fruits, plants, and seeds provided for our sustenance. "And on the banks, on both sides of the river, there will grow all kinds of trees for food. Their leaves will not wither nor their fruit fail, but they will bear fresh fruit every month, because the water for them flows from the sanctuary. Their fruit will be for food, and their leaves for healing." (Eze 47:12) Then in conclusion, we find in Revelations 22:2, the following vision. "...through the middle of the street of the city; also, on either side of the river, the tree of life with its twelve kinds of fruit, yielding its fruit each month; and **the leaves of the tree were for the healing of the nations.**"

Even though we will touch upon knowledge so profound that in the ancient world it was only given to High Priests, I want to affirm that the plant kingdom's gift of healing is freely part of our natural symbiosis. It is already actively supporting your life, and you have experienced it in many delightful ways.

Plants are critically important to life on earth. They are the foundation on which all life stands. The botanical kingdom is a vast chemical factory, which interfaces between light and dark, sun and earth, drawing energy from each and synthesizing it into molecules of carbohydrates, proteins, and fats necessary to all other forms of organic life. Plants provide the "crude fuels" which all animals and humans break down to produce ATP (adenosine triphosphate), our high-grade fuel. More than that, these 'factories' of life shape and sustain an environment capable of sustaining all organic life on earth.

Within plants there are essential oils, which are the high-grade fuel making this miracle possible. When we bring their pure essence into our lives, we too acquire the ultimate goodness plants have to offer...which, in many ways, is the fountain of life. I believe this was the understanding that the ancient High Priests and perfumers celebrated as they took great care to extract and prepare oils worthy of anointing in the name of Spirit. They called their art 'alchemy', and what alchemists had to say about themselves and their beliefs reveals much about the results to which they were so devoted. For an alchemist, every particle of creation had three parts—a body, soul, and spirit. Their chemical art involved dissolving the physical essence with which they were working and then allow the soul and spirit to purify itself and re-condense into quintessences of the rarest form. With regard to essential oils, they would distill over and over again until the final products were highly potent medicines.

The value of essential oil to the constitution of plants (and by extension to us) is not merely for the aroma it provides. There is a vital force encoded within these 'essences', which insures the plant will be protected, healed, restored when damaged, and propagated when conditions allow. One of their main functions in the plant is to heal all wounds and defeat invasion. They are also the world's most powerful anti-oxidants. From the beginning, at the very foundation of life, was the means to safeguard life and assure its continuance and expansion. This protection, which is extended to all the rest of life, is perhaps the most extraordinary contribution of plants. So amazing is it that it touches every level of our existence.

There is a circle of life that is ever widening. This

applies not to a species, but also within a single member of a species, and even within a single cell. Every life entity has a beginning. It grows, protects itself, and replicates itself. When this circle is unbroken there is a state of integrity we call 'wholeness'. In a state of wholeness, life can continue, grow, and evolve. Ultimately, wholeness is the secret to health, and interestingly, smell is the signatory quality that informs all of nature instinctively about the health of its members and the wholeness that supports them.

Many healers, from mainline to alternative, have reported certain aromas (odors to be more accurate) related to certain diseases, and then reported the disappearance of the odors as healing progressed. A fascinating diagnostic tool that is being explored today, and with great success, involves training dogs to respond in certain ways to particular body odors. Their ability to diagnose cancer and diabetes in early stages that other more "sophisticated" systems have not detected is simply phenomenal.

A joyful, knowledgeable, and skillful use of aroma can provide one of the most important of all healing tools. This is partly because of the constituents in plant essences, and also partly because we are hard-wired to respond through our sense of smell to seek the essences that will assist us in our needs for wholeness. This is true, whether it happens to be nutrition, healing, or emotional reparation. The right smell can effectively lead us to what we need, or stimulate a state of wholeness where disease and unhappiness cannot easily enter.

Countless memories, and rich sensations of being alive, are indelibly connected with our recollections of smell. How many times, before sipping fresh squeezed orange juice, have you paused to inhale the fragrance and felt a surge of nourishment even before it touched your lips? How often have you been cheered by the smell of fresh baked cookies and felt satisfied without ever consuming a calorie? I still remember from my childhood, the fondest memories related to smell: car trips from my hometown into Fort Worth were always enlivened by passing Mrs. Beard's Bakery! Trips to my uncle's ranch were rich with scents from fresh baled hay to barnyard aromas, which were not altogether offensive, because I associated them with the happy events of gathering eggs and riding horses. To this day, those scents make me happy!

Remembrance of such experiences provides the basic understanding and power behind why aroma therapy is so effective and sacred oil blends have such power upon our consciousness.

Aromas can have a powerful effect on all levels of your being: body, mind, emotions, and spirit. A vital, living fragrance can directly affect everything about you, from how you feel, to your motivation for living, to your actual lifespan.

Of all five senses, our sense of smell is the only one directly linked to the limbic lobe of the brain, the emotional control center. Anxiety, depression, fear anger, and joy all emanate from this region. The scent of a special fragrance can evoke memories and emotions before we are even consciously aware of it. Where smells are concerned, we react first and think later. All other senses (touch, taste, hearing, and sight) are routed through the thalamus, which acts as the switchboard for the brain, passing stimuli onto the cerebral cortex (the conscious thought center) and other parts of the brain. Therefore, all our other senses are to some degree 'filtered' by the various conditions of 'conscious allowance'.

Much more will be revealed in later chapters about how to use essential oils to access these hidden memories. However, as we begin, I want to impress upon you how the power of even a subtle aroma can affect your state of consciousness. Scent embraces and infuses our life both consciously and unconsciously. Knowledge of how to use it for our betterment is the foundation of aroma therapy.

This book will not be limited to sacred oil blends used for anointing, or even to essential oils, because the subject of scent belongs to nature and does not lend itself to being labeled and limited. Scent is not the property of our intellect, but a powerful force that defines our experiences of life. Once we grasp the ancient and indelible relationship we have with scent, we can then appreciate how we are innately affected by it whether we are being anointed for healing or making a full sensory dive into a beautiful pink grapefruit. That realization also impels us to believe that the ultimate therapeutic gift that plants and their aromas may offer us is a 'therapy of wholeness'.

In considering the wholeness of scent, I am reminded of St. Paul's letter to the Philippians (4:18), in which he remarks, "I am amply supplied, having received of Epaphroditus the gifts you sent. They were a fragrant offering, well pleasing to God." Most likely the use of the word 'fragrant' was a metaphor referring to the endearment they contained rather than some aromatic oil. His statement is a potent reminder that spiritually we are just as attuned to our senses as we are physically.

Our soul does not form its plans and goals as we would a corporate agenda, because our soul unfolds its purposes with a greater sense of wholeness and intuitive evolution. Even so, it has deeply seated aspirations which form the imprint of our lives. These aspirations can and do represent a kind of orientation and conscious intention, which then causes the outer manifestations of our life.

Does our soul or spirit actually exude or 'smell' aroma, or does the body provide this sense for the soul's pleasure? I am not sure. What I do know is that poetic associations through the ages have used scent to suggest a bridge between conditions of the soul and a corresponding scent. To wit: the sweet aroma of Heaven, the stench of betrayal, the bitterness of self denial, the freshness of an open mind, and so forth.

In my experience, there are a number of vital similarities between the way we are nurtured, guided, and protected by our basic physical needs **and** our highest spiritual nature. Both are instinctive and empathic. Both serve without reservation or condition. This is quite unlike our normal cognitive functions and behavioral patterns, which are conditioned, encumbered, often focused on fragmented parts of our life (especially the parts under challenge), and frequently resistive to change.

By creating positive associations between our favorite scents, which directly affect us physically, and a corresponding spiritual (or higher mental) state, we can create a bridge that passes over the troubled water of many life challenges. While there are challenges that must be met immediately and head-on, most of our troubling situations are just murky waters created by causes beyond our control or by others with whom we have confused our feelings. In those cases, we can turn our attention toward self nurturing. We can re-establish our wholeness while the outer situations are working out their tangles and revealing a clearer picture of what further can be done.

This is a type of wholeness therapy which I sometimes refer to as a 'Conspiracy of enlightenment and wellness'. I call it that because we are eliciting the soul's greater knowing and sensitivity which sees few if any limitations. Then we engage it with the innocent, base-level knowing of the body, which is hard-wired to seek protection and healing in the most effective way. In our ancient history, smell was the body's highest survival sense. It was so vital that it is the only one of our five ordinary senses having a direct connection to the autonomic nervous system, without any conscious filters or permissions. By connecting our highest faculty (the heart and soul) with smell, our most primal initiatory sense for well being, we are by-passing all the sludge and confusion in between, which could misdirect us or pin us down. The principle is that by moving us up to the soul's radiance, under the authority of love, we will reconstruct our wholeness in the gentlest, most beautiful and effortless way through our body's inner knowledge.

To do this, we first attend to the physical and emotional needs of our bodies, whether that would be to provide rest, therapy, play, or more desirable work. Use good sense to move conflicts aside. Then use good **scents** to fully engage your body in what you are doing! That would include everything from a summer peach exploding with aroma while the sweet nectar cools your throat, to more frequent enjoyment of natural fresh air, to the selection of essential oils that uplift and enrich your spirit, to anointing with a special oil blend in a moment of greater reverence. All of these wonderful aromas wake up the autonomic nervous system and create signals of well-being on a deep cellular level that cannot be screened out by the cognitive mind or overwhelmed by environmental turbulence. While doing this, turn your attention to the aspirations of your soul. These could be plentiful and unique for each person. However, in his teachings to me, Jeshua offered seven aspirations that are constant desires of the soul. They are: Innocence, Compassion, Abundance, Wisdom, Peace, Forgiveness, and Joy. Whether you choose to focus on one of these primary aspirations, or another that has special power and meaning in your life, as you connect it with scent, you engage your body and soul in a primal nurturing and uplifting. Wonderful changes can occur (and remain) as to seem miraculous.

Our soul's aspirations are always guiding us toward fulfillment or moving us around the roadblocks to it. Usually, though, we are so focused on the affairs of the world that we do not see this higher work, or utilize its great benefits. By acknowledging our spiritual aspirations, and specifically putting our attention on them, we bring them into all levels of conscious living and even our unconsciousness patterns. The process of awakening is an ever-widening circle, and wherever you are in the circle is a wonderful place to be. Sometimes it can be temporarily challenging as you "blow through" a bit of resistance or old limiting beliefs, but it is always relieved by the brighter view on the summit of that experience.

It is very healing to create a direct association between an aspiration of the soul and an aroma you are moved by emotionally. In doing this you have performed your first practical application of anointing. There may be different occasions for anointing, but there is only one universal reason for it. That is to establish an unimpeachable connection between body and soul that **your senses can recognize.** This is true, whether one is using a blend of oil steeped in sacred tradition or one that is the fruit of modern inspiration. When this vital connection happens it is always sacred, even if the application was a casual one. The sacred connection is more important than which fragrance or oil blend are used. Jeshua gave me formulas that coordinate profoundly and universally with the aspirations of the soul, but they are not the only ones that can uniquely trigger the association for you. There will be more on that to come.

For now, let's apply this knowledge to having a delightful experience. Aroma therapy is simple and joyful, and you can continuously explore ways of connecting with your favorite natural aromas. The next time you shop for fruits or vegetables, smell them before making a selection. Let your nose tell you which ones are most nourishing, or at least most likely to support your needs. You will instantly feel better for it, and also have more nourishing food.

Here is a wonderful and simple home spa aroma experience that can begin in the grocery store. For this you will need to choose a delectable, fragrant piece of citrus fruit, a cucumber, a few buds of clove, and some green tea. On returning home, chill the cucumber and set aside the clove and green tea. Take your piece of citrus fruit, lemon, orange, or grapefruit, and hold it close to your nose. Breathe deeply. Now step outside and hold it for a moment. Continue to breathe deeply with your nose close to the fruit. Notice how the oxygen, nitrogen, and other gases in the atmosphere have accelerated the aroma. Enjoy the energy that this simple natural experience provides.

Next take your piece of citrus fruit and peel the rind. Put the peelings in a pot of boiling pure water and enjoy the aroma it adds to your home. Chill the fruit for later. After a short while add more water if necessary and a few buds of clove. This will accelerate the experience, and you'll learn why in the next chapter. This bestows a natural bouquet of aromas into your home, which will bring vitality instead of allergic reactions and headaches as room deodorizers often do. There is no substitute for the energy of LIFE! Next, add a bag of green tea, turn off the heat, and let it steep.

While the tea is steeping, draw a bath, and slice two thin pieces of cucumber to place over your eyes while in the tub. Add the entire elixir of citrus, clove, and green tea to your bath water, and cover your eyes with the cool cucumber. As you delight in the aromas of your warm bath, you can enjoy eating your chilled fruit. This is a spa experience of exceptional delight, all provided by the bounty of nature. Enjoy the aromas and all the sensations of warmth and coolness on your eyes. Just relax and let nature do its healing work.

On another occasion take a piece of fruit, such as an apple, with you on a walk. Be sure to inhale it as you munch away, and notice the increased vitality you get from the whole experience. If you work out in a gym, try taking fruit instead of an energy bar (which is loaded with carbs), and smell your way to energy instead of just consuming calories. I especially like to take apricots in season and open them to smell the kernel, which is rich with natural B17 (Laetrile). I think you will be amazed with the difference it makes to also inhale your natural refreshments. If it does not smell good to you or give you an immediate energy boost, chances are it has no vitality in it. There is no better way of selecting fresh fruits and vegetables than to smell them before putting them in the grocery sack! Actually, you can have a good nourishing experience for free by just walking through a farmer's market where produce has been grown naturally and picked ripe. Smell and enjoy! The bounties of life and fragrance are all around you.

Chapter 2

What are Essential Oils?

We call them "essential" because they are the life blood of plants. They carry the plant's archetypal imprint and convey it into every cell and chemical process. All cellular chemistry and growth in the plant kingdom is through a binary process of substances either held or suspended in water, or held and suspended in lipids (oil). These two alternating groups are responsible for all the cellular structure, growth, health, and life of a plant. Water carries vital nutrients and is the medium of exchange in all of a plant's life processes. The lipids hold the blueprint of what makes each plant unique and what provides its defenses in life as well as how its DNA plans to propagate and survive. In short, the lipids are the Vital Essence of any plant. Most essential oils are antimicrobial to some extent, since one of their main functions in the mother plant is to heal all wounds and defeat invasion. Because these essences evolved symbiotically within nature for the purpose of healing, they never damage healthy tissue or create auto-immune reactions within their host plant. Inside our own bodies essential oil is gentle as well. It promotes healing, unlike harsh synthetics that can actually cause tissue damage and scaring.

Essential oils are composed of tiny molecules weighing less than 500 atomic molecular units (amu). By comparison, other fatty oils weigh more than 1000 amu. The miniscule size of essential oils allows them to pass through all the tissues of the body and into every cell within minutes of contact. Essential oil can pass through any cell wall, and it takes only one molecule of the right kind to open a receptor and communicate with a strand of DNA. Only molecules less than about 800 amu can cross the blood-brain barrier. Therefore, essential oil can go where very few other substances can reach. This is aided by the fact that there is nothing in essential oil to trigger the highly guarded immune defense system protecting the brain's membrane. Another rapid conductive factor is that lipid molecules are more transdermal than water soluble ones.

Therefore even inhaling a small amount of essential oil can have a profound effect on the body, brain, and emotions. Sometimes too many oil molecules can overload the receptor sites and they freeze up without responding at all. Therefore, one must be very cautions with excess quality. Less is more. One drop of essential oil contains approximately 40 million-trillion molecules, which is enough to cover every cell in our bodies with 40,000 molecules.

Modern scientific research has shown that there are several reasons why essential oils can improve our health. More recent studies have shown that they have amazingly high antioxidant properties. We are all familiar with the importance of having enough antioxidants to fight the harmful free-radicals that damage our cells and slowly cause us to age and develop chronic degenerative diseases. We know that fruits and vegetables are rich in antioxidants, and among them, berries have among the highest contents of antioxidants. Scientists at tufts University have developed a scale for the US Dept of Agraculture called the ORAC Scale: Oxygen Radical Absorption Capacity. The higher the score the more capable any food or topical substance is of destroying free radicals. The free-radical fighting ability of antioxidants is measured in ORAC units. Broccoli and spinach have ORAC values of 890 and 1,260 respectively. The berry group (blueberry, strawberry, raspberry, and others) has ORAC scores of between 1,200 and 2,400 (highest in blueberry). And, the superstar of berries, which is the Ningxia wolfberry or *gou-ji*, has ORAC value of over 25,000. It is also very rich in life-force.

Even beyond that, essential oils, rank as the world's most powerful anti-oxidants. The best fruits do not come close to the ORAC power of essential oils. The weakest of essential oils (sandlewood) has an ORAC value above 2,000. Lavender essential oil has ORAC value of nearly 3,700. Lemon essential oil is over 6,000, lemongrass nearly 18,000; cinnamon bark over 100,000; and, amazingly, clove essential oil has ORAC power of over 10 million! With that kind of capacity to knock out harmful free-radicals, we should not be surprised at all that essential oils can heal.

Essential oils have long been shown to have antiseptic, antiviral, antibacterial, antifungal, and anti-parasitic properties. These have been validated by recent scientific studies and have given rise to safe, natural alternatives to chemical drugs in the fight against microbes and other infections.

Apart from being able to trap harmful oxygen free-radicals, essential oils have the unique ability to use the oxygen molecules to help transfer nutrients across the cell walls, into the cells, and even into the cell nuclei. Thus essential oil mops up harmful radicals while at the same time enabling the cells to feed and become healthier and stronger to withstand any further damage as they go about their normal functions.

The most fascinating of all discoveries about essential oil, with regard to human and planetary health, concerns their electromagnetic frequencies. These frequencies can be measured in every life form. New equipment developed by Bruce Tanio, Head of the Dept. of Agriculture, at Eastern Washington University is now being used at Johns Hopkins to study the frequency of substances, food, and the frequencies associated with human health and disease. Their measurements on the human body found that a healthy person has a frequency around 62-68 MHz. When a person's frequency dips to 58 MHz, cold symptoms can manifest. Flu symptoms start at 57 MHz, Candida at 55 MHz, and Epstein Barr syndrome at 52 MHz. Cancer can begin when the body falls below 42 MHz. The process of dying begins at 25 MHz and goes to zero at death. The frequencies of essential oils are between 52-320 MHz, the highest of all known organic substances. The highest is Rose at 320 MHz. By comparison fresh herbs measure 20-27 MHz, dry herbs 12-20 MHz, and fresh produce 5-10 MHz. Processed or canned food measure zero. They may contain chemical nutrition if not adulterated by additives, but there is no vital life force nutrition.

History of Healing with essential oils

Aromatherapy is one of the most ancient healing methods. It is the science of utilizing aromatic essences extracted from plants for health and healing. The natural essences are used to balance and harmonize the energies that operate within us, and promote the health of the body, mind, and spirit. Although the term *aromatherapy* was not used until the 20th Century, the use of essential oils goes back thousands of years, its origins usually being attributed to Ancient Egypt and India.

Pure essential oils are painstakingly distilled from flowers, seeds, shrubs or other parts of the plant and kept in special containers since the oils are volatile. Because the resources (mostly flowers, herbs, seeds, and spices) have always been readily available, aromatherapy has been practiced by all cultures for the duration of recorded history. It is said that essential oils were the first known medicines. The Chinese may have been one of the first cultures to use aromatic plants for well-being. Their practices involved burning incense to help create harmony and balance. India is probably the only place where such knowledge has been continuously in use without interruption. Ayurevedic medicine, which uses essential oil for healing, is the oldest continuous form of medicine in the world. The Vedas, which is the central and sacred book to this tradition, codifies and uses fragrances for liturgical as well as therapeutic purposes. It mentions over seven hundred different healing essences, including sandalwood, myrrh, cinnamon, spikenard, and ginger.

This tradition is said to have supplied knowledge to the perfumers of Egypt. When King Tut's tomb was opened in 1922, it was reported that 350 liters of essential oils were found. Many ancient Egyptian scrolls contain various prescriptions using essential oils. In ancient times it was a commodity more precious than gold, and was often exchanged as gifts between kings and emperors. The oils and their uses are also mentioned many times in holy books, especially in the Bible.

The early Egyptians used mainly infused oils and herbal preparations for spiritual, medicinal, fragrant, and cosmetic use. It is thought that the Egyptians coined the term *perfume*, from the Latin *per fumum* which translates as "through the smoke." Egyptian men of the time used fragrance as readily as the women. Later, the Egyptians invented a rudimentary distillation machine that allowed for the crude extraction of cedar wood oil. It is also thought by some that Persia and India may have also invented crude distillation machines, but very little is known.

The Greeks learned a great deal from the Egyptians, but Greek mythology apparently credits the gift and knowledge of perfumes to the gods. The Greeks also recognized the medicinal and aromatic benefits of plants. Hippocrates, commonly called the "father of medicine," practiced fumigations for both aromatic and medicinal benefit. A Greek perfumer by the name of Megallus created a perfume called Megaleion, which was a blend of myrrh in a fatty-oil base. It was used for several purposes including its aroma, for its anti-inflammatory properties on the skin, and to heal wounds.

The Roman Empire built upon the knowledge of the Egyptians and Greeks. Discorides wrote a book called De Materia Medica that described the properties of approximately 500 plants. It is also reported that Discorides studied distillation. Distillation during this period, however, focused on extracting aromatic floral waters and not essential oils.

A major event for the distillation of essential oils came with the invention of a coiled cooling pipe in the 11th century. Persian by birth, Avicenna invented a coiled pipe which allowed the plant vapor and steam to cool down more effectively than previous distillers that used a straight cooling pipe. Avicenna's contribution led to greater use of essential oils and exploration of their benefits.

Within the 12th century, an Abbess of Germany named Hildegard grew and distilled lavender for its medicinal properties.

Within the 13th century, the pharmaceutical industry was born. This event encouraged great distillation of essential oils.

During the 14th century, the Black Death hit and killed millions of people. Herbal preparations were used extensively to help fight this terrible killer. It is believed that some perfumers may have avoided the plague by their constant contact with the natural aromatics. A famous blend of clove, lemon, cinnamon, eucalyptus, and rosemary was developed in 15th century England, according to the legend by four thieves, who used these and other aromatics to protect themselves while robbing plague victims.

Within the 15th century, more plants were distilled to create essential oils including frankincense, juniper, rose, sage, and rosemary. A growth in the amount of books on herbs and their properties also begins later in the century. Paracelcus, an alchemist, medical doctor, and radical thinker is credited with coining the term "Essence" and his studies radically challenged the nature of alchemy as he focused upon using plants as medicines.

During the 16th century, one could begin purchasing oils at an "apothecary," and many more essential oils were introduced. It continued for the next four centuries as a kind of "grass roots" medicine, or medicine of the common man.

Modern day aromatherapy owes its renaissance mainly to the work of the French. Among them was Dr. Rene-Maurice Gattefosse, who accidentally discovered the healing power of lavender oil in his cosmetic laboratory. He had plunged his burnt hand into the oil thinking it was water, and was surprised to see rapid healing. He continued to apply the oil until it healed, leaving no scar at all. During World War II, his colleague, Dr. Jean Valnet, used essential oils to fight infections when his antibiotics supply ran out, and saved many lives. After the war, Dr. Valnet and his students did further research and found that essential oils have powerful anti-infective capabilities, improve the immune system, and also enhance the delivery of nutrients into the cells. Since that time, much scientific evidence has been accumulating about the reason for these healing successes.

Aromatherapy for Emotional Well-Being

Aromatherapy may assist, sometimes greatly, with particular emotional issues. Additionally, the proper use of essential oils may enhance a person's emotional outlook and provide support and help to maintain balanced emotions during the day.

Because of their miniscule size and volatile nature, essential oil molecules can affect us profoundly just by inhaling them. From the back passages of the nose, they travel directly into the brain to a central part called the amygdala. This is the headquarters of the limbic system, which the oldest part of our nervous system (biologically speaking). This part of our brain stores, files, and manages all emotional experiences, and it does so without relating that sensory data to words, thoughts forms, or any consciously formed concepts. Smell is our most primal non-verbal sense, which also provides a profound, often unconscious link to our emotions. Sound is another primordial perception that goes directly into the amygdala. Thus, there also is a legendary connection between emotion and music.

Again, I will remind you to be alert to the holistic nature of our sense of smell. Memories of smell, like emotion, are neither fragmented nor even centralized, but diffused throughout your whole being. What I am about to tell you is both shocking and confirming of that assertion. Medical and psychological research has now provided conclusive evidence that while the center of the brain is the coordinator of emotional memories, the actual memories **are not stored there.** The amygdala is a receptor, cataloger, and dispatcher of memories, but the memories are stored in other parts of our body, especially in cases where the emotional experience is too overwhelming or traumatic to assimilate in present time. All experiences received directly through the amygdala—primarily emotions, smell, and sound—will be assigned to some other part of your body to retain until you are ready to deal with it. Perhaps it will just stay there as an indelible part of how you see yourself or respond to life. A perfect example is a favorite song from your youth that you hear and all at once your whole body goes into rhythm.

The amazing thing about our bodies is that each one is composed of over 100 trillion cells, within which is a strand of DNA capable of storing up to six gigabytes of memory. Because of this the, any part in your body can store feelings, sensory experience, and emotional memories delegated to it by the emotional brain. The total memory capacity in every human body is greater than **all the computers in the world.**

When stored emotions interfere with positive survival signals to our cells and organs, or even worse, when they give distorted signals, illness can result. Because the stored emotions are below our conscious awareness, we are most often not even aware that this is happening. For example, an emotional upset during a meal, which was also accompanied by the smell of maple syrup, may be stored in the stomach to alert the stomach to protect itself in the future from any further instances with maple syrup. That sounds absurd, but in the days when humans were hunters and gathers, that smell might have been a poison berry not yet "officially" known as a poison. This type of automatic interplay between emotion, sensation, and reaction was part of a biological learning process controlled by the amygdala as we evolved and accumulated experience. Today, of course, we can override that function with conscious understanding, and even use our conscious mind to clean out many useless and possible destructive memories.

Often these unconscious memories are reacting to environmental stimulation without our knowing. This mechanism can certainly interfere with conscious living and even be destructive. Take, for example, the incident with maple syrup. The stomach's association between eating it and becoming stressed may prevent the person from ever digesting it again without problems. In the worst of cases, that stressful memory stored in the stomach could eventually result in ulcers or other disease. This would be true for any part of the body where the Amygdala had assigned and forgotten a challenging memory.

Scent often triggers emotions that correspond to the memory stored in an area of disease or distress. This can be beneficial or disastrous, depending on whether it is happening unconsciously or being therapeutically addressed. Through skillful use of scent it becomes possible for us to remember and deal with forgotten emotional memories.

Essential oils give us a way of accessing the non-verbal portion of our constitution where feelings and emotions are stored. Keep in mind that emotional associations, both positive and negative, have many variables. For example the scent of roses may remind you of your first romantic kiss in a garden, or the roses at your grandmother's funeral. Not all fragrances provide the same level of benefit for all persons. You are unique, and part of what makes you special is the blueprint of your emotional nature and your emotional memories. Past memories associated with particular aromas can have a positive or negative effect. Therefore, rely on your instinctive intelligence as your guide to what fragrance is right for you in any given moment or circumstance. Do not force yourself to use any oil that elicits negative feelings or that you don't like.

Citrus oils such as grapefruit, sweet orange, and lemon provide a good first experience with essential oil. The clean, refreshing smell of citrus oil helps provide an immediate connection with flavors you have enjoyed. Inhaling them brings emotional balance and a more positive outlook. They are wonderful to use alone or in a blend with lotions for those times when you need an invigorating lift.

The pulse points of your neck or wrist are the perfect places for applying light, invigorating fragrances such as citrus. For most therapeutic treatments, however, the soles of your feet are the ideal place for applying essential oils, because your feet have a more tolerant protected surface and yet the structure of the foot is a map of the whole body. Most of the anointing in the Bible was on the feet, and the washing of feet was usually a preface to that sacred gifting.

I have included a list for you below of pure essential oils most commonly recommended by aroma therapists to assist with emotional issues. In keeping with the holistic orientation of this book, I have also included aromas in each category that you might easily find in your kitchen or back yard as well as pure essential oils. It is important, however, that you treat this list only as a starting point. Experiment within the confines of safety, and utilize fragrances that bring about the result you seek.

Anger: Jasmine, orange, patchouli, roman chamomile, rose, ylang ylang, bergamot, myrrh, marjoram.

Anxiety: Rose, sandalwood, bergamot, cedar wood, clary sage, frankincense, geranium, orange, lavender, mandarin, patchouli, roman chamomile.

Concentration: Cedar wood, cypress, basil, myrrh, lemon, peppermint, rosemary sandalwood, yang ylang.

Confidence Grapefruit, jasmine, orange, rosemary, bay laurel, bergamot, and cypress.

Depression: Bergamot, clary sage, frankincense, geranium, grapefruit, jasmine, lavender, lemon, mandarin, neroli, orange, roman chamomile, rose, sandalwood, and ylang ylang.

Disappointment: Frankincense, clary sage, ginger, cypress, juniper, orange, geranium, sandalwood, spruce, rose, thyme.

Fatigue, exhaustion, and burnout: Basil, bergamot, black pepper, clary sage, cypress, frankincense, ginger, grapefruit, jasmine, lemon, patchouli, peppermint, rosemary, sandalwood, and vetiver.

Fear: Bergamot, cedar wood, clary sage, roman chamomile, frankincense, grapefruit, jasmine, lemon, spruce, orange, and sandalwood.

Guilt: Frankincense, roman chamomile, cypress, juniper, lemon, geranium, sandalwood, spruce, rose, thyme.

Grief: Rose, sandalwood, cypress, frankincense, neroli, and vetiver.

Happiness and Peace: Bergamot, frankincense, geranium, grapefruit, lemon, dogwood, orange, rose, sandalwood, ylang ylang

Insecurity: Bergamot, cedar wood, frankincense, jasmine, sandalwood, African violet, and ginger.

Irritability: Lavender, mandarin, neroli, roman chamomile, and sandalwood, and black pepper.

Loneliness: Bergamot, rose, clary sage, frankincense, roman chamomile, and vanilla.

Memory and Concentration: Basil, lavender, cypress, hyssop, lemon, peppermint, rosemary

Panic and panic attacks: Frankincense, lavender, Bergamot, myrrh, and rose.

Resentment: Jasmine, rose, tansy.

Restlessness: Frankincense, angelica, bergamot, lemon, geranium, sandalwood, spruce, rose.

Stress: Grapefruit, vanilla, bergamot, rose, sandalwood, ylang ylang, clary sage, frankincense, geranium, jasmine, lavender, mandarin, patchouli, and roman chamomile.

Chapter 3

The History and Use of Sacred Oil blends

When we speak of Heaven on Earth, our minds call forth incredibly beautiful images of life in a state of near perfection, even with its complexity, diversity, and challenges for growth, because it is whole. The physical, emotional, and spiritual powers of life are seamlessly integrated. The evocation of that state, and all the healing power that comes with it, is the purpose of anointing with sacramental blends of essential oil.

Sacramental blends are called that because all stages of their growth, harvesting, distilling, and blending have been treated with reverence for the life within them and the life they have to offer. There is a special devotion of effort that exceeds normal standards of agricultural and manufacturing quality. It extends into the realm of spiritual guidance, inspiration, and experience concerning the art and science of healing and blessing with essential oil.

Because of the inspirational and healing power of scent, we can only imagine the reverence that was held in the ancient world for rare blends and elixirs that could change life in miraculous ways. Indeed, they were more costly than gold. In the hands of skilled and sensitive 'perfumers' (as they were called in those days) blends were created which alchemically transmuted single plant essences to even higher energetic levels. What a miraculous blessing. It was truly believed to be a gift from God, and indeed it is.

When Moses established the priesthood and was preparing to consecrate Aaron and his sons, God instructed him in the protocol of sacred anointment. Moses was told to take exact and specific proportions of myrrh, cassia, calamus, cinnamon, and olive oil and make them into a sacred blend for consecration. He was then told to anoint the tent, altar, and all the instruments of consecration, *"so they will be most holy, and all that touches them will be holy. Anoint Aaron and his sons and consecrate them so they may serve me as priests. Say to the Israelites, This is to be my sacred anointing oil for generations to come."* (Exodus 30: 22-33). Anyone who used the mixture inappropriately or divulged the secret blend to those not qualified to know it would be exiled from the tribe. This sacred oil was a symbol of God's presence among them and the sacred bond that made the people one people, under one leadership. Thus, it follows throughout the Old Testament with the anointing of kings and priests. In the Twenty-third Psalm, King David writes, "Thou anointest my head with oil. My cup overflows." This is perhaps the most quoted verse out of 156 mentions in the Bible of sacred anointment.

The Bible is full of references to herbs, fruits, plants and seeds provided for our sustenance, beginning in the first chapters of Genesis. In addition to hundreds of references to plants, nuts, and seeds for food and medicine in the Bible, there are mentions of 33 aromatic species of plants and more than 1,000 references to the use of essential oils. This is because essential oils were in daily use by the Israelites, indeed, all people of the ancient world. More importantly, fragrance was used to mark the vital passages of life—its beginning, its end, and the important attainments along the way. Birth, marriage, initiation into positions of authority and leadership, ordinations into priesthood and kingship, and finally embalming of the body at death were all marked and celebrated with fragrant oils. We see this in the life of Christ, beginning at his birth with the present of Myrrh and Frankincense from the Wise Men; the times he was anointed or anointed others; and finally at his tomb on Easter morning when Mary Magdalene arrives to prepare his body with oil.

In the New Testament we see all points in the life of Jesus anointed with oil. It began at his birth with the present of Myrrh and Frankincense from the Wise Men. During his ministry he was personally anointed or anointed others in many instances. On two occasions during his final week preceding crucifixion, copious amounts of costly essential oils, including spikenard and myrrh, were poured over him. (Matthew 26:7, 12: Mark 14:3; and John 12:3-8).

As part of his ministry, Jesus taught his disciples about the spiritual art of anointing to bring about healing with oils (usually olive) which were infused with precious spices and aromatic essential oils. *"And they went out, and preached that men should repent. And then cast out many devils, and anointed with oil many that were sick and healed them."* (Mark 6: 12-13) It is also clear that they did not assign a medicinal value to the oil in the sense of matching herbal chemistry with specific ailments. Therefore, it is unlikely they were practicing aroma therapy as a treatment technique. Rather, they were infusing an event or a situation with the signatory presence of "wholeness." This was conveyed in a living way by sacramental blends, which were believed to convey the presence of the Holy Spirit. The confirming evidence of that is that it wasn't always oil used for this conduction of Spirit. They knew, as Jesus had taught, that it is faith under the power of Spirit that actually heals. In one instance, probably for the lack of oil, Jesus simply used spit and mud to anoint the eyes of a blind man before he was healed.

Study of the Apostles as they spread the Gospel reveals that sacred oil continued to be a crucial part of their healing ministry. In the book of James, the inspired writer exhorts: *"Is any among you sick? Let him call for the elders of the church; and let them pray over him, anointing him with oil in the name of the Lord; and the prayer of faith shall save him that is sick, and the Lord shall raise him up."* (James 5:14, 15)

This reminds us to respect the ultimate meaning of what it means to anoint, which in a sacred context, is to fill with Spirit or convey Spirit. Not every anointing involves the use of oil. Often, anointing is directly from Spirit through other forms of blessing. However, it is notable that the term anointing, even in ancient times, is virtually synonymous with the use of some sacramental oil blend. This is because essential oil is actually the life essence, or spirit, of plants. As we have seen in the previous chapter, these essences have the highest energetic resonance of any other natural creation. Moreover, the rare and exquisite fragrance created by blending aromas can suggest a non-material presence with an even higher resonance and greater evocation of Spirit than any one species of plant could ever emit on its own. Biblical records about sacred oils almost always are referring to blends. There are, however, a few exceptions where single precious oils are appropriate for an occasion.

One poignant account in the Gospels of Mark (14:3) and John (12:3) tells us about Mary Magdalene anointing Jesus with oil to prepare him before his arrest. *"Then Mary took a pound of ointment of spikenard, very costly, and anointed the feet of Jesus, and wiped his feet with her hair: and the house was filled with the odor of the ointment."* There were those who rebuked her for wasting so much perfume equal to a year's wages. But Jesus replied, *"Why are you bothering her. She has done a beautiful thing to me. The poor you will always have with you, and you can help them any time you want. But you will not always have me. She did what she could. She poured perfume on my body beforehand to prepare for my burial. I tell you the truth, wherever the gospel is preached throughout the world, what she has done will also be told in her memory."* When one considers how much he cared for the sick and the poor, it becomes obvious how sacred was the experience of being anointing with precious oil.

Healing and Wholeness

The recognition of wholeness and its unique place in the flourishing of life is as old as it is modern. In our most advanced sciences today, the subtle demarcation between chaos and order is of great importance, and a great deal of study has been devoted to observe and determine when and how chaos turns into order and vice-versa. One thing is fairly constant, however: a preponderance of chaos will shred any remaining vestiges of prior order. And, a preponderance of order will protect itself from chaos by forming an integrated wholeness capable of repelling chaos! I believe it was this recognition of how life works that inspired the first creations of "Wholeness Oils" or Holy Oils. These oils represented the wholeness of the plant. It is then conveyed into other forms of life as a continuing, sustaining force, symbolizing and actually IGNITING wholeness by contagion of positive effect.

It is in the tradition of anointing for purposes of spiritual blessing that we refer to some rare essential oil blends as sacred. However, in doing so we acknowledge that it is the Spirit within and the Spirit guiding our actions which is sacred. To convey this spiritual blessing we use oil blends that connote spiritual presence for celebrating special moments of attainment, acknowledging our wholeness, or responding to a call for healing when wholeness seems to be broken.

We find this not only in our Judeo-Christian traditions, but in traditions from all over the world. Hippocrates, the father of medicine, states that "the way to health is to have an aromatic bath and scented massage every day." As far back as the fourth century BC he recognized that burning certain aromatic substances offered protection against contagious diseases and this is a method we can adapt to social gatherings today for the same reason, but with the advantage of specific scientific information about the antibacterial and antiviral properties of particular aromatic oils. Indeed, the history of fragrance needs to be reevaluated in the light of our modem knowledge and the protective and health-giving properties of aromatic substances.

One might think that aromatic fragrances were used in early times to cover up bad smells caused by lack of sanitation and hygiene, but that is highly unlikely. Ancient texts and archeological discoveries reveal that that early civilizations were as concerned with cleanliness as we are. In 5000 BC the people of the city of Mohenjo Daro, in modem Pakistan, were heavily focused on cleanliness. Archaeologists found a communal bath measuring 39 feet by 23 feet in addition to wells in every house. The Egyptians took personal hygiene seriously, as shown by the earliest recorded recipe for a body deodorant in the Papyrus Ebers of 1500 BC. The Egyptian priests used aromatic substances not only for embalming their Pharaohs but also in their role as physicians for treating manias, depression, and nervousness. Many of the oils used in ancient Egypt came from China and India, where there is evidence to suggest they were already in use for a thousand or more years before the Pharaohs.

It is logical to assume that these oils were used in varied ways, sometimes for mundane pleasure, sometimes for specific ailments, sometimes for celebration, but most of all for holy occasions. I should also add at this point that what we call essential oil today is the product of steam distillation, a process that did not exist in ancient history. Steam distillation makes possible a very potent extraction of the plant and also to eliminate the various toxic byproducts that could also be present. Steam distillation is what made aromatherapy, as we know it, possible by creating very pure substances that can be studied as to their effects on specific ailments. In the ancient days, mostly what was called precious oil was created through infusions of carrier oil (such as olive) and the source of some precious element, much the way we put fresh tarragon in olive oil to have a gourmet dressing. This leads me to believe that most of the anointing, healing, and celebrating in the ancient days was carried by the mystical and majestic power of "Wholeness" and the Holy Spirit.

This is confirmed by the ancient Greeks, who had a very high opinion of aromatics, attributing sweet smells to divine origin. In ancient myths, gods descended to earth on scented clouds, wearing robes drenched in aromatic essences. The Greeks believed that after death they went to Elysium where the air was permanently filled with a sweet-smelling aroma which came from perfumed rivers. And in Roman as well as Greek bath houses, aromatic oils were extensively used, as prescribed by Hippocrates, for health.

The Babylonians went so far as to perfume the mortar with which they built their temples—an art they handed down to the Arabs who built their mosques in the same aromatic way. In India the early temples were built entirely of sandalwood, ensuring an aromatic atmosphere at all times. Clay tablets from Babylonia dating from around 1800 BC detail an import order which included the aromatics of cedar wood, myrrh, and cypress, all used as oils therapeutically today.

What is common to all forms of healing and blessing is to envelope the recipients in a safe and nurturing space. That kind of safe space can be created or provided in many ways from a nurturing home, to a temple retreat, to a hospital room, to a nature sanctuary, or a better state of mind and heart. Through the healing cocoon, we are offering the appropriate care and respect necessary to repair any broken wholeness and initiate the process of healing. It can begin with kind words, a compassionate heart, and a knowledgeable, understanding mind. Now, let's include in that range of healing possibilities an encompassing aroma that knits together body, soul, and emotions. In all these ways and more, what we are creating is a temple of healing.

All religions and spiritual practices have focused on some sort of temple or place of sacred congregation. The temple was the focus of community and a powerful symbol for its "Wholeness." Usually, these temples took the form of architecture or some other exact and specific place where communities could join to celebrate or practice their common beliefs. This naturally caused the temple to be a target for conquering forces, and the history of ancient people (even modern nations) is full of anguish and grief over the destruction of temples and holy places. Many have been rebuilt, and others never will be.

An imperishable Temple

Two thousand years ago mankind was on the edge of embracing a larger awareness about who we are. In light of this readiness, Jesus brought into consciousness and practice, a revolutionary new idea...of a temple that could not be destroyed once it was fully established. This was the idea of individual wholeness, in attunement with universal wholeness. To that end he taught about atonement and spiritual fulfillment. He preserved the idea of a community temple or sacred place, but for him the fundamental prototype of every temple was the Sacred Heart, a place central to every human body, mind, and soul where one's connection to God is everlasting. With this profound invitation to humanity to return to its divine connection with the Creator's a new covenant was proclaims. That new covenant was for the rebuilding of the most ancient of all temples...the one within, where in true sanctuary man could be in a complete state of love with God and love of others as himself. He saw this instatement of wholeness as our ultimate responsibility on the planet, in caring for ourselves and others. The Apostle Paul was teaching this wondrous truth when he asked the people of Corinth, "Know you not that you are the temple of God, and that the Spirit of God dwells in you?" Co 3:16.

This is a temple not built with bricks and mortar, but with consciousness and a caring heart. It first involved clearing of old stagnant consciousness focused on judgment and negativity through acts of forgiveness. That clears the way for a positive infilling—with new aspirations of the soul that are attuned to physical, mental, emotional, and spiritual unity. In a state of wholeness we become vessels of the living God. The heart would be the altar in this temple. In Jesus' original conversations with me in 1992, he told of seven aspects or dimensions of higher intelligence that may be found within the Sacred Heart. They are Unity, Love, Life, Respect, Honesty, Justice, and Kindness. Each dimension successively develops the principles of love and unity. Through this, one's connection with our Creator is eternal and ever expanding.

As part of this process we respond to and employ these higher dimensions of intelligence. A desire is born for greater wholeness within our self and among those with whom we share life. These desires are primal, and since they are directed toward wholeness, they extend beyond all goal boundaries in a very unconditional way. Jesus referred to these desires of the heart as sacred aspirations. They represent the trigger points within our consciousness that bring forth memories of wholeness and make it a greater passion than any condition or activity that fragments us. A sincere desire to be whole again, with ourselves, with God, and with others is the key to atonement or at-one-ment. Most certainly atonement is the key to the temple about which Jesus spoke.

If you listen to the teachings of the heart, you will find there is great simplicity to the temple within. Figuratively speaking, there are six pillars with a floor and a glass-domed, light filled ceiling. The pillars are compassion, forgiveness, innocence, peace, joy, and abundance. Compassion is not love because of something. It is love beyond all things. Forgiveness is not to "get" something, but rather to release something—most especially one's pain, fear, and judgment. Innocence is not because one has never "erred," but because an inner core of goodness allows a person to know when he or she has. Peace is not when one successfully brings order to the world, but when order has been brought to one's self. Unlike happiness that is bound to pleasure and needs for positive reward, joy is the soul's exhalation regardless of circumstances. Joy is when the soul celebrates being not of the world yet a blessing to it. Abundance is not the prosperity of material acquisition, but the realization of infinite supply that requires no attitudes of scarcity, hoarding, or greed. The foundation on which all of these pillars stand is Wisdom. That is the guiding aspiration, encompassing all possibilities, sometimes called Sophia or the Divine feminine virtue. When all of these unconditional states of being are focused into active service for living, the presence and light of Christ shines forth through and from the Temple. The ultimate aspiration for wholeness is our desire to resume our own intimate relationship with Divinity, thus discovering the Christ light within ourselves.

An interesting characteristic of this Temple is the natural rapport that exists between it and the soul and also between it and the body. The human condition and all of its emotions, mental states, and agendas seem to be the real source of disassociation we feel about our personal Temple. As we look in this direction for a model of greater wholeness, it also becomes a trigger point for memories of the soul and yearnings of the body. This is how anointing with oil can sew a flawless seam.

According to the covenants of higher consciousness, revealed by Jesus, we are our own priests and priests to one another. Therefore, we are all entitled to use anointing oils on ourselves and to administer them to others. We are all ordained by the Holy Spirit for this. Not only are we all endowed with the spiritual and temporal duties of ministering to ourselves and others, but we also have responsibility for our own wellness through right living and right thinking. The primary and most important temple in which each of us must worship and find God is the temple of our own soul. It is in that temple, and no other, that we must ultimately find union with our Creator. "Ye are the temple of the living God." (II Corinthians 6:16)

Historically there were five types of anointing:

❖ The act of anointing signified consecration to a holy or sacred use; hence the anointing of the high priest

(EX. 29:29; Lev. 4:3) and of the sacred vessels (Ex. 30:26). The high priest and the king are thus called "the anointed ones." (Lev. 4:3.5.16; 6:20; Ps.132:10). Anointing a king (or leader) was equivalent to crowning him (1 Sam. 16:13; 2 Sam. 2:4). Prophets were also anointed (1 Kings 19:16; 1Chr. 16:22, Ps. 105:15).

❖ Anointing was also an act of hospitality (Luke 7:38, 46). It was the custom of the Jews to anoint themselves with oil, as a means of refreshing or invigorating their bodies (Deut. 28:40; Ruth 3:3; 2 Sam. 14:2; Ps. 104:15). Some Arabs still continue this custom today.

❖ Oil was used also for medicinal purposes. It was applied to the sick, and also to wounds (Ps. 109:18; Isa. 1:6; Mark 6:13; James 5: 14).

❖ The bodies of the dead were sometimes anointed (Mark 14:8; Luke 23:56).

❖ To call forth and recognize the higher anointing of the Holy Spirit. Jeshua, as the Messiah was called the "Anointed" one (Ps. 2:2; Dan. 9:25-26), because he was anointed with the Holy Spirit (Isa. 61:1) figuratively the "oil of gladness" (Ps. 45:7; Heb. 1:9)

Why was anointing done?

❖ To bring anything or anyone into greater wholeness. To consecrate a person, object, or location to God or to its highest use: Webster's definition of consecrate is "To devote irrevocably to the service of God." God instructed Moses to consecrate the tabernacle, utensils and priests by anointing them (Ex. 40: 9-11, 13,

47

15). As living temples of God, we can use our bodies and possessions to honor God. By anointing them, we consecrate them to serve their highest intended purpose.

❖ It was part of the healing process: To the followers of Christ, anointing with oil was part of the ministry to the sick. James 5:14 says, "Is any one of you sick? He should call the elders of the church to pray over him and anoint him with oil in the name of the Lord." Mark also mentioned this practice was used by the disciples, who "drove out many demons and anointed many sick people with oil and healed them" (Mark 6:13).

Who can anoint people?

We tend to think of anointing being a sacramental act that only priests, mystics, and those solely dedicated to God can perform. But, this is a misconception, installed by some traditions of religious hierarchy. Even in the New Testament we see that anyone can perform this loving blessing: "And behold, a woman in the city who was a sinner, when she knew that Jesus sat at the table in the Pharisee's house, brought an alabaster flask of fragrant oil, and stood at his feet behind him weeping; and she began to wash his feet with her tears, and wiped them with the hair of her head; and she kissed his feet and anointed them with the fragrant oil. (Luke 7:37-38) The Bible even records self-anointing: "So David arose from the ground, washed and anointed himself and changed his clothes; and he went into the house of the Lord and worshiped." (2 Samuel 12:20)

When to anoint:

- ❖ Before prayer, meditation, or worship. (2 Samuel 12:20)
- ❖ After cleansing ourselves: "Then I washed you in water; yes, I thoroughly washed off your blood, and I anointed you with oil." (Ezekiel 16:9)
- ❖ To pull ourselves up after realizing and repenting misdeeds, misunderstandings, or failure. (2 Samuel 12:20)
- ❖ Prior to going into a competitive situation that it may serve the greatest good and lead to true victory. (Isaiah 21:5, 2 Samuel 1:21)
- ❖ When someone is sick (Mark 6:13, James 5:14)
- ❖ When we need protection (Isaiah 21:5, 2 Samuel 1:21)
- ❖ When preparing to serve God in a special way (Isaiah 61:1; Exodus 40:13)

What to anoint: People, places, and things were anointed throughout the Bible. Here are some suggestions of things to anoint:

- ❖ People (family members, friends, anyone who asks.)
- ❖ Buildings (house, office, rooms, church, schools)
- ❖ Possessions: Beds (especially if there are disturbing dreams or sleeplessness), computer, monitor, TV, VCR, furniture, cars, professional equipment.

What to use for anointing: Fragrant oil of the highest quality is the traditional substance for anointing. Other substances can and have been used, although we tend to think of something precious. This is because the

49

significance of anointing is directed toward sacred reunion, which is empowered by the spiritual reason behind the anointing. That is both an open-ended and powerful statement, which leads us first to pay attention to cause, the calling, and the vehicle of inspiration.

In his years of teaching and counseling me, Jesus has led me to create special blends of anointing oils to strengthen our resolve with regard to the key aspirations that connect and focus our body, mind, and soul. These oils are highly recommended, which are dedicated to sacred reunion, are discussed in the Appendix. In addition to their beauty, the greater value of each blend is that it addresses a particular aspiration of the soul. I have found invariably in my work that one or more of these aspirations are part of the reason for restoring wholeness, and thus for anointing. They may be intuitively selected as part of giving oneself, or another recipient, an invitation to seek and accept that blessing.

There are also ancient sacred blends, and pure essences that strike a cord with the purpose or reason for anointing. Always the relevant truth and higher guidance should be consulted. Prior to using oil or any other substance, we ask God to bless it and use it as a holy medium for the highest good.

Where, on the body, to anoint:

❖ The crown of the head for sacred ceremony, spiritual blessing, or spiritual invocation. This is most appropriate for the Christ blessing.

❖ The forehead for inspiration, mental clarity, greater foresight. This is appropriate for either the blessing of innocence or wisdom.

❖ Base of the throat for speech, expression, creativity, social engagement, and verbal commitments. This is appropriate for either the blessing of joy or abundance, depending on the occasion.

❖ Heart area for emotional clearing and for healing illnesses with great emotional content. This is most appropriate for the blessing of compassion.

❖ Solar Plexus for self esteem, confidence, and physical stamina. This is appropriate for either the blessing of joy or abundance.

❖ Lower back for vitality, physical cleansing, relaxation, and general recuperation after any challenging situation or project. This is appropriate for the anointing of peace.

❖ The hips for striding forward with any project or aspiration. This is a wonderful place for the blessing of abundance.

❖ The knees for flexibility (mind, heart, and body)

❖ The ankles for standing in one's own power.

❖ The bottoms of the feet for reaching all organs or ailments of your body. There is a whole map of your body on the bottom of your feet. You might want to consult an acupressure chart for these exact points. Anointing the feet, especially after a warm foot bath, is an expression of great caring that can initiate immediate healing responses. The three lower points, knees, ankles, and feet are especially powerful for the blessing of forgiveness.

What to say when you anoint:

"Through the power of God, the love of the Holy Spirit, and the generosity of natural life I offer this blessing. May it awaken and strengthen the purpose to which it is dedicated. May it uplift, inspire, and heal whatever is hurt and needing love. May the power of love and the oneness of spirit use this sacramental blessing for the restoration and protection of life. Give us wisdom to accept and to live in that wholeness."

While you speak the above words, lightly wet your fingertip with oil and touch the person or object with it.

Chapter 4

How to use essential oils and Sacred Oil blends

It is important to understand that the three-pronged subject of scent, essential oil, and sacred oil are united through our own instinctive intelligence, which seeks for wholeness and recognizes it in life. Through scent, we are drawn into this unity, and through the fragrant oils we are able to celebrate it!

Learning this subject is a little like learning any new language. First you accumulate some basic elements of understanding, and then you gain more certainty with it as you use it and experience the connections it can provide between yourself and others. Finally, we explore and enjoy the language until it becomes an extension of our consciousness.

The goal is to recover your sense of smell in the fullest and most vital way as a natural expansion of your life. Explore, enjoy, and develop a sense for what aromas bring you to life, and what they mean to you. Continue to grow in your understanding of food aromas; celebrate your personal life with fragrances that express your inner beauty; and allow any sacred oil blends you use to help define and deepen your moments of reverence. All of life is sacred; therefore, any essence of life can bring us into a deeper understanding of our place in its wholeness.

In this chapter is a sampling of practices and recipes for using sacred oil blends, essential oils, and even fresh fragrances from life. By becoming actively involved with the ones that appeal to you, it will stimulate a deeper understanding of how we are healed, enlivened, and made more joyful by our immersion in the aromas of life.

One of the most satisfactory aspects of using essential oils spiritually, therapeutically, and cosmetically is that they enter and leave the body with great efficiency, leaving no toxins behind. The most effective way to use essential oils is by external application or inhalation. The methods used include inhalation, body oils, lotions, compresses, baths, hair rinses, perfumes, room sprays, and a variety of room diffusers. Although, under qualified supervision, some essential oils can be orally ingested, this is in fact their least effective use, because it requires that they pass through the digestive system. There, they come into contact with digestive juices and other matter affecting their chemistry. Unlike chemical drugs, essential oils do not, as far as we know, remain in the body. They are excreted through perspiration, and exhalation, urine and feces. Expulsion takes about three to six hours in a normal, healthy body.

Remember that a little goes a long way. Sometimes too many oil molecules can overload the body's receptor sites, causing them to freeze up without responding at all. Also, even the purest of oils can sometimes cause sensitivity when applied directly to the skin, especially in large amounts. Therefore I recommend to always pre-test your tolerance and not to exceed that level. Putting a little oil in your lotions or carrier oils can be a good way of introducing essential oil to your body. Your body's acceptance and tolerance will grow as it resolves "issues" that may have caused initial sensitivity. If there is any sensitivity at all, begin with a room diffuser until your body, mind, and emotions have assimilated the impact of a particular fragrance.

The soles of your feet are the ideal place for applying essential oils directly, because here the body has a more tolerant protected surface and yet the structure of the foot is a map of the whole body. Most of the anointing in the Bible was on the feet, and the washing of feet was usually a preface to that sacred gifting.

Room diffusers can be as simple as an object or sculpture on your desk that you anoint daily with your favorite oil. Sometimes I place a drop on my jewelry. Other ways to experience the aromas are by applying it to a cool light bulb before turning on the light, or simmering a few drops in a small pot of water. This water can then be added to your bath water later in the evening or used for a hair rinse. Enjoy the interplay between your sense of smell and your intuitive intelligence. Each day, allow your instinctive response to lead you to a fragrance that empowers and uplifts your spirit. Follow your guidance through prayer, meditation, and creative yearning to reach for that which will strengthen the temple and inspire the betterment of your day. The purpose of Sacred Oils is to uplift your consciousness, enhance your spiritual practices, and abundantly enrich your life.

These are some of my favorite applications:

Fragrance:

Because essential oils contain no alcohol, their scent clings within one or two feet of your body, in the "zone of intimacy". This way you will have the benefits of an exquisite fragrance and share it discretely with others. One or two drops are all that is necessary. Place it on your pulse centers at the throat or wrists. For a more overall fragrance that is still subtle, add a few drops into your body lotions. In their pure state, essential oils are both volatile and absorptive into the skin, so there is little residue to be picked up by clothing. I have never seen clothing permanently stained by it. In fact, rather large spills I have made while bottling were completely "gone" from my slacks the next day due to the volatile nature of pure oils.

Make your own perfume

- ❖ Your favorite Sacred Oil or other essential oils
- ❖ Pure high-proof Vodka. Do **not** use wood alcohols which you buy in stores and pharmacies as they are poison to your body.
- ❖ Distilled Water

To make your perfume, mix at least 25 drops total of essential oils with 2 1/2 ounces of alcohol. Shake for a few minutes, and then let it sit for 48 hours (or up to 6 weeks- the longer it sits, the stronger the smell). Add 2 tablespoons distilled water, stir, then pour through a coffee filter and put it in a bottle.

Body splashes:

These are scented waters that can be splashed on or sprayed for toning, uplifting, or relaxing. Use the same technique as with perfumes, but dilute them further so they give off a light and gentle aroma. They are easy to make and make wonderful presents for friends. Have an array of them in your bathroom, and use them as your mood requires. They do a great job of making you feel good without leaving an oily residue.

Personal spritzes and room fresheners

Once you have your perfume, it's a quick step to make your spritz. Just dilute it further with distilled water and put it in a spray bottle where it's handy for a pick-me-up.

Scented hair

Apply 2 drops of your chosen essential oil to the bristles of your hairbrush and brush your hair well. The oils will leave your hair with a wonderful aroma.

Lotions:

Just add a few drops to your lotions and creams. Then shake or stir them well. You may have to shake or stir them again with each use because lotions are generally emulsions of oil **and** water, so the oil you add may separate. This varies, however, with different lotions.

Sacred Oil soap

- ❖ 5 ounces glycerin soap
- ❖ 1/4 teaspoon Sacred Oil
- ❖ Bronze and gold mica dust
- ❖ Ultra fine gold fabric glitter
- ❖ Oval soap mold

Melt the soap. Stir in the Sacred oil and Gold mica dust. Pour into 2 molds. Allow them to set and then un-mold when their firm. You may keep them indefinitely by freezing in a zip-loc bag. To make a special gift, you may add a light dusting of the gold glitter. If you've frozen the soap allow it to thaw and warm before adding the glitter or wrapping.

Emotional release: This application is primarily for affecting the emotions. It requires a small piece of cotton, about the size of a Q-tip end. One or two drops of oil is put onto the cotton ball, and this is placed in the ridge of the RIGHT ear (not the left), just above the opening to the ear, NOT INSIDE THE EAR. The reason this is so effective is that the five main cranial nerves form a juncture or ganglia at this point. The essence is absorbed through the skin and has an immediate effect on one's state of mind and emotion.

Home spa treatments with Sacred Oil and essential oil

Baths: Nothing is more relaxing than a long hot soak in a scented bath. Hot water releases the essence of oils so that its fragrance can be inhaled with the steam of the warm water, while your skin takes it in as nourishment. Plus your whole bathroom will smell wonderful for hours! Experiment with the right amount for you. Five to eight drops should be sufficient, depending on the size of your bath tub. A few drops are also great in your Jucuzzi or sauna.

Foot bath: Add two to four drops to a bowl of warm water. Soak your feet for twenty minutes and then apply scented massage oil to keep in the warmth.

Bath and massage Oil: Most essential oils mix well with unscented carrier oils such as sweet almond, olive, jojoba, and safflower. Organic unscented oils can be purchased in any health food store.

Here is a well-balanced oil blend for most skin types. It is nourishing and soothing and it is not too heavy or light. It provides an excellent base for an essential oil or Sacred Oil blend. This oil blend may be used directly on the skin for massage or you may use two teaspoons in your bath water for an uplifting aromatic experience.

- ❖ 1 1/2 oz. olive oil
- ❖ 3 oz. almond oil
- ❖ 1 oz. sesame oil
- ❖ 1 oz. canola oil
- ❖ 1/2 oz. wheat germ oil
- ❖ 15-30 drops essential oil of choice

❖ 1 oz. basic bath and massage oil blend or other carrier oil of choice

Pour the oils in a jar, cap with a tight fitting lid, and shake well. You can create a wide assortment of aromatherapy oils for the bath by adding essential oils to the basic oil blend or to any other carrier oil of your choice. These oils can be used for both bath and massage.

Relaxation

This blend is for relaxation and stress relief. It will induce a deep relaxation of the tissues, muscles and joints, and re-establish a good energy balance.

Blend the following essential oils into one ounce of basic bath oil. Massage as desired or use as bath oil.

❖ 3 drops Lavender
❖ 3 drops Tangerine
❖ 3 drops Marjoram
❖ 1 drop Chamomile

Eucalyptus oil

Eucalyptus is an effective analgesic which is often used to relieve muscle, nerve, and joint pain. Apply massage oil to the affected area before a warm bath, and then massage the area again after your bath. I like a blend of Lavender and Eucalyptus for even better results. When massaging small areas like a shoulder you can double the amount of essential oils used.

Hot rock massage

This is a spa treatment from the Arizona desert. Select a large, flat smooth stone, the size of your palm. Heat a stone in a low temperature oven until warm through and through, but not too hot to hold comfortably. Rub some scented massage oil into the stone and use this heated rock to give your partner a soothing massage. The heat from the stone relaxes and penetrates the muscles. Use up to 15 drops of essential oil per 1 oz. of unscented oil. Start with less drops, you can always add more.

Bath salts

- ❖ 1 cup sea salt
- ❖ 1 cup Epsom salt
- ❖ 1 cup baking soda
- ❖ Your favorite essential oils
- ❖ You'll want about 6 drops of essential oils per 1/4 cup salt blend
- ❖ Use 1/4 cup per bath. This makes enough for several baths.

Relaxing lavender honey bath

Honey has a calming effect on our body. Combined with pure essential oil of lavender it's a sumptuous bath treatment.

- ❖ 2oz. of honey
- ❖ 5 drops lavender

❖ Combine in a jar.
❖ Use 1-2 Tablespoons per bath.

Lemon citrus soak

Lemons have been used for hand and nail care for centuries. Lemon Juice and the essential oil of Lemon whitens nails while stimulating healthy growth. Try this Refreshing Citrus Soak

❖ 8 oz. spring water
❖ 1 Tablespoon Aloe Vera Gel
❖ 10 drops Lemon oil
❖ Mix and soak fingertips for 10 minutes.

Rosemary mist

This bracing, stimulating mist is a superb post-shower, after you've toweled off but skin is still a bit damp. In spray bottle place 5 ounces distilled water, 1 tsp olive oil, 6 drops rosemary essential oil and 1 sprig fresh rosemary. Shake well to mix and spritz on as desired.

Cornmeal face scrub

Essential oils can be incorporated into many facial products. This facial scrub is very invigorating.

❖ 1/4 cup yogurt
❖ 1/4 cup cornmeal
❖ 15 drop of Oil of Joy or Oil of Aliveness
❖ Mix together and refrigerate a couple of

❖ Hours before using. Store in the refrigerator.

Ginger body scrub

❖ Use this one in the morning as the essential oils are invigorating.
❖ Sea Salt 1/4 Cup
❖ Cornmeal 1/4 Cup
❖ Olive oil 1/3 Cup or another base oil.
❖ Ginger 2 drops
❖ Peppermint 4 drops
❖ Rosemary 3 drops

Mix salt and cornmeal. Combine warmed oil and essential oils then mix with dry ingredients. Use in the shower or standing in the tub. Apply in circular motions, working from the extremities inward, working towards the center of the body and the heart. Rinse with warm water. Gently pat dry. Your skin will feel smoother and have a nice glow.

Fragrant bath fizz

❖ 1 cup baking soda
❖ 1 /2 cup cornstarch
❖ 1 /2 cup citric acid
❖ 15 drops essential oil

Mix all ingredients in a bowl. Add food coloring to a small amount of the mix in a separate bowl. Add colored mix to remaining mix and blend. Mist the salts with a mister enough so that they hold together but not enough to start fizzing. Pack these salts into a soap mold. Flip over onto a piece of waxed paper and allow the molded fizzies to dry overnight.

Buttermilk bath salts

- ❖ 1 cup buttermilk powder
- ❖ 1 cup Sea Salt Add
- ❖ Up to 24 drops of essential oils.

Blend well and keep in a sealed jar. Use 1/2 cup per bath. This makes enough for 4 baths.

Bath mush

- ❖ 1/4 cup aloe gel (the pure kind from the health food store)
- ❖ 1/4 cup honey
- ❖ 1/4 cup sea or rock salt
- ❖ 1/4 cup heavy cream or powdered milk
- ❖ 2 teaspoons jojoba oil (optional)
- ❖ 5 drops essential oil

This is a blend made right before the bath. It's not as messy as you think, but you have to stir it well when you pour it into the bath water to make it disperse. It leaves the skin feeling soft, smooth, and very nourished.

Bath cookies (For bathing, not for eating)

- ❖ 2 Cups Rock Salt
- ❖ ½ Cup Baking Soda
- ❖ ½ Cup Cornstarch

❖ 2 Tablespoons Almond Oil
❖ 1 Teaspoon Vitamin E Oil
❖ 1-2 Eggs, 6 Drops Essential Oil

Mix together and pat out on waxed paper. Then cut with a cookie cutter in the shape you want. Bake at 350 degree 10 - 12 minutes. Allow to cool. Use 1-2 per bath. Keep these in an air tight container and don't plan to store them indefinitely because of the eggs. They make great gifts.

After bath toner

❖ 2 oz. green tea
❖ 5 drops lavender essential oil
❖ 5 drops geranium essential oil

For a very refreshing treat up this bottle of green tea and essential oils to balance the pH of your skin after cleansing. Place the ingredients in a glass bottle. Essential oils do not dissolve in water or tea so be sure to shake this mixture well before each use to make sure the essential oils are dispersed. Use a cotton pad to apply to face and neck area after cleansing.

Aromatic body powder especially for the feet

❖ Mix 1 cup cornstarch, 1 tablespoon baking soda in a jar with a tight fitting lid.
❖ Add 15-20 drops of your favorite essential oils.
❖ Shake well.

Spa Chocolates

For an exquisite treat for body, heart, and soul, essential oils can be infused into chocolates or any other sweets by placing the loose chocolates in a box then adding a piece of absorbent paper to which you have placed 1 drop of essential oil. Cover and let sit until absorbed, a few days should do it. Among the Sacred Oils, I would suggest Compassion or Joy. Try other oils like Orange or Mandarin for a different twist. These can be eaten...YUM!

Some old stand-bys for aroma health remedies

Essential Oils for Cold and Flu

Some of the best choices in anti viral oils are ravansara, eucalyptus, and tea tree, which help fight viral infections and support the immune system. Mix 10 drops in 1 tablespoon carrier oil and massage upper chest and back, or place 3 drops on a tissue and inhale and inhale as often as needed.

Essential Oils for Congestion

Eucalyptus, rosemary, lavender, and tea tree oil loosen congestion. They help fight viral and bacterial infections, while providing a little stimulation to your whole system. Mix 10 drops in 1 tablespoon carrier oil and then massage the upper chest and back, or place 3 drops on a tissue and inhale as often as needed.

Cold and Flu Fighter

- ❖ 4 drops Sweet Eucalyptus
- ❖ 4 drops Scotch Pine
- ❖ 3 drops Lemon

Add to a large bowl of steaming water. Covering your head, lean over the bowl and inhale deeply for several minutes. This combination may also be added to a diffuser or vaporizer.

Germ Fighter Spray

Here is an antiseptic, germ fighting spray to use on cuts and scrapes. It is also good to spray on your hands after washing to prevent the spread of illness among our family members and close associates. It may also be used as a room spray to inhibit the spread of air born contagion.

- ❖ 12 drops Tea Tree
- ❖ 6 drops Eucalyptus
- ❖ 6 drops Lemon
- ❖ 2 oz. distilled water

Combine ingredients and add to a spray bottle. Shake gently before each use.

Essential Oils for Headache

For headaches use peppermint, lavender, or roman chamomile. Put 1 drop of essential oil on each temple and at the nape of the neck. Or mix 5 drops of Lavender and 1 drop of Peppermint into 1 Tablespoon carrier oil or lotion and massage neck and shoulders.

Essential Oils for Body Aches

Lavender, Roman chamomile, and sweet marjoram help to soothe aches and pains. Mix 10 drops of essential oil in 2 Tablespoons of carrier oil or lotion and massage areas of discomfort.

Four Thieves

Here is a legendary blend for health protection that you can recreate at home. It's a blend of clove, lemon, cinnamon, eucalyptus, and rosemary oils. The story is that four thieves in 15th century England used this blend to protect themselves while robbing plague victims, hence the name.

Fragrance for your home:

Humidifiers

Add 1 to nine drops to the water container, then run as normal.

Light Bulbs

Add a few drops to a cool light bulb and then turn it on.

Diffusers

There are many devices that can be used to diffuse essential oils. Some are made specifically for that purpose, such as the cold diffusers with a fan that distribute aromas saturated into a filter pad. Some are heated by a candle flame. But any non-porous object can be the anointed recipient of a few drops of oil. The natural volatile nature of the oil will eventually fill a whole room with sweet fragrance.

Incense

The primary purpose of using incense is to cause the oil to become ignited. This process releases properties that cannot be released in any other manner. An easy way to create incense is to use self-igniting charcoal tablets. Put a few drops of oil onto the unlit tablet, and then light it with a long match, being careful not to burn your fingers. Once a small section of the tablet is lit, then you can place it in a heatproof dish. It will continue to burn. Relax and enjoy. This method is excellent for meditation and prayer.

Scented Beeswax Heart

Scent a room with this decorative accent. Use a cookie cutter to cut a heart shape from a sheet of natural beeswax. Wrap the heart in cheesecloth and infuse it with a few drops of Oil of Compassion. Place the wrapped heart in a plastic bag for a week. Remove and discard the cloth and glue a ribbon hanger to the back of the heart. You can even decorate it with dried flowers and a bow. Hang it anywhere you plan to be!

Ice Candles

Melt one pound of paraffin in a double boiler. Cut a milk carton to height desired, center a taper candle inside. Then fill with crushed ice. Add six drops of your favorite Sacred Oil and a sprinkling of glitter to the cooling paraffin.....pour the paraffin into the carton. Let cool, then pour off the water and tear away the carton to reveal a candle that glistens like ice and smells like Heaven.

Aromatic Rainbow Rocks

- ❖ 1/2 cup plain flour
- ❖ 1/2 cup salt
- ❖ 1/4 teaspoon essential oil (your favorite scent)
- ❖ 2/3 cups boiling water
- ❖ Food coloring, if desired

In a bowl, mix all the dry ingredients well. Add essential oil, and boiling water to that mixture. The scent will be strong, but it will fade slightly when dry. For colored stones, add food coloring, one drop at a time until the desired shade is reached. Blend thoroughly, and form balls into different shape and sizes to look like stones. Allow them to dry, and than place the "rocks" in a bowl or dish to scent a room. A nice alternative to potpourri!

Sachet

Add a few drops of any of the Sacred Oil blends to cotton balls and enclose them in a pillowcase, which can then be laid among your clothes. This will help keep unwanted pests from enjoying your clothes.

Scented Stationary and wrapping paper

Make your personal letters and greeting cards extra special. Place 1 drop of any Sacred Oil on the inside corner of each card. Seal and send as usual. This way you can send a blessing of sacred scent across long distances.

Other practical uses of essential oil in your home

Orange glass shiner

Use orange glass shiner to polish any glass or mirror to a lovely finish and shine. It leaves your room smelling fresh and wonderful instead of chemical.

- ❖ 4 ounces water
- ❖ 4 ounces apple cider vinegar
- ❖ 1 tablespoon borax
- ❖ 1 tablespoon orange essential oil
- ❖ 1 teaspoon lemon essential oil

Blending Procedure: Combine all ingredients in a heavy duty plastic spray bottle and shake well before each use. Spray on glass or mirror and wipe immediately with a clean cloth. The shiny surface will emerge. Stubborn stains like old toothpaste glop and chewing gum come off with ease, plus the aroma is pleasant and uplifting. It's best to use gloves with this cleaner and remember to shake before using the evenly incorporate the essential oils. As with all household cleaners, keep this one out of the reach of children.

Dishwashing liquid

Lift your spirits while washing the dishes. This is not suited for automatic dishwashers.

- ❖ 10 drops Lemon essential oil
- ❖ 10 drops Lavender essential oil
- ❖ 10 drops Orange essential oil
- ❖ Liquid castile soap or other mildly scented dishwashing liquid.

Fill a 32oz. squirt bottle with liquid soap and add the oils. Shake well.

Kitchen sink and counter-top scrub

- ❖ 1/2 Cup Baking Soda
- ❖ 1/8 Cup Vinegar
- ❖ 5 drops Lemon essential oil
- ❖ 5 drops Orange essential oil
- ❖ Combine all ingredients

❖ Try Lime or Bergamot also.

Potpourri

You can make your own potpourri using plant materials such as whole flowers, petals, leaves, pine cones, and wood chips. The very best way to dry your own flowers and plant material is to use a dehydrator. This not only speeds up the drying process, but the natural fragrance of the flowers and plant material is often retained. It also helps preserve the shape of the flowers and drastically reduces the likelihood of mold occurring as you dry your items. Even inexpensive dehydrators work quite well. An easy way to find fresh flowers and other items suitable for drying is to check your own flower garden or back yard. Ask your local florist to save flowers with broken stems, and other items that they can't sell. They will sell them to you inexpensively. Roses with missing petals are great for potpourri because you can pluck all the remaining petals, dry them, and turn them into potpourri. To dry potpourri in a dehydrator, trim and clean your flowers, and petals, place them in the dehydrator carefully so the items don't touch each other. The type of material that you are drying, the air humidity and your brand of dehydrator will all contribute to the length of time it will take to dry your potpourri materials. Dry the material until it is thoroughly dry, otherwise mold can occur. Flowers and petals should feel crisp. It is best to allow your items to cool before determining whether they are done. Be sure to follow all safety and usage instructions for the model of dehydrator that you use. If you are planning for a spicy potpourri, in a separate process or on a different shelf you can include very thin slices of apple that has been marinated in spice such as cinnamon or nutmeg.

After the batch is dry and thoroughly cooled, mix together your desired assortment of flowers, petals, leaves, and wood chips. I suggest a glass or ceramic bowl to display your potpourri as the essential oils can absorb into porous surfaces. Using a dropper or the orifice reducer that is built into your Sacred Oil bottle, sprinkle 5-8 drops of your blend onto your potpourri. Based on the strength of the chosen blend and the amount of your potpourri materials, you may need to adjust the number of drops that you use. When the aroma weakens, add more drops of the blend to re-freshen the aroma.

Some Common Sense Precautions

Essential oils, including Sacred Oil blends, are for aromatic and topical use only, to facilitate a higher state of mental, emotional, and spiritual well-being. They should never be taken internally. Pure essential oils are many times more potent than perfume, and should not be used liberally on the skin without first testing for tolerance in a small area or diluting with a neutral carrier oil or lotion. There are times when a qualified aroma therapist will direct a client to take an essential oil internally. However, these instances would be limited to oils from edible herbs and plants, such as cumin, oregano, and garlic, and would be taken only in small amounts, and singularly. Oil blends, even from edible plants, are not recommended for internal use simply because the stimulation and reactions may be too complex to monitor. Digestive fluids may also cause chemical changes in the oils and result in unwanted chemical byproducts that could be stressful to the liver and kidneys. This does not seem to be a problem when oil is assimilated through the skin, providing moderation is used and care is exercised to determine personal sensitivity. Keep it away from your eyes and be sure to avoid mucous membranes, where sensitivity is extreme.

Keep your oils stored in a cool place away from sunlight. Keep them tightly closed, as pure essentials are volatile and will evaporate if left open to air.

Keep the oils away from children or anyone else who does not know to respect their potency. Be particularly careful if you are pregnant or have any other sensitive medical condition. Be sure and consult your physician before using essential oils if you have any health questions at all.

Essential oils are not safe for topical application to cats. The terpineols in all essential oils pose an elimination problem to a cat's special liver physiology. Inhaling diffused aromas in the room seems to be tolerable for them. In fact, cats are often attracted to the aromas and receive therapeutic benefits from them. Just be sure, after applying oil to yourself that you wash your hands before stroking kitty. Dogs and horses have a similar tolerance to oils as humans, although their olfactory receptors are so much more powerful than ours, undiluted oils could be overwhelming to them. Please consult a holistic veterinarian before applying an essential oil to any animal.

If you have any specific plant allergies, such as to cedar, it may be no different with cedar oil. The possible exception to this may be that you are only allergic to cedar pollen. In that case, the oil may be perfectly tolerable to you. Experiment. Essential oils are so compatible with the human constitution and supportive of it that most people have nothing but positive experiences with essential oils. Just respect your own sensitivities and never force yourself to use anything that your better judgment dictates against. If any redness or irritation develops, discontinue that particular oil or use it in greater moderation. Everyone is a unique snowflake of individual possibilities, pattern, and sensitivities. Providing you observe the above precautions, using moderation and common sense, a thoughtful use of essential oils for personal well-being fits perfectly within the healing maxim of Hippocrates to "First do no harm." They are a great first line of defense on behalf of health and wholeness. They provide a wonderful ladder toward the higher realms of emotional and spiritual elevation.

Appendix

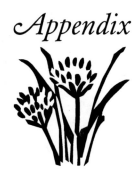

The Temple Fragrances

The original eight Sacred Oil formulas that Jeshua gave to me were to be used for remembering and restoring the wholeness of our own personal temples. Therefore, we call them the "Temple Fragrances."

As with all sacred oil blends, these blends are the result of chemical transformation. By that, I mean that the whole is something much more than the sum of the parts, and virtually represents a new and greater essence than any separate component would possess. Through higher guidance, intuition, and skill, the ingredients were selected for their unique property and value, but even more so for their botanical susceptibility to symbiotic union into a greater whole. For an essential oil to qualify for use in a Sacred Oil blend it must be absolutely pure. Just as there are different grades of diamonds (and true investment grades are not available commercially) so, too, there are many grades of essential oils. These qualities are determined by a number of factors. Among these factors are such things as the quality of the source plant (whether it was commercially grown or wild harvested) and the manner of its refining. Most especially, care and understanding must have been given to every step of its preparation. Not only is this necessary to extract and preserve the fragrance, but also to retain its life essence thereafter. The Temple Oils are blends of the purest oils available, and in most cases, from wild harvested plants. They were grown, harvested, and lovingly processed by people whose traditions for preparing sacred oil runs deeper than the pages of history. These particular formulas have been developed under the direction of Jeshua to promote the greatest value for spiritual, mental, and emotional elevation as we restore the Temple of our Lives. Many times their effects are miraculous.

Christ Scent is a blend using many of the ancient sacred oils including myrrh, frankincense, and sandalwood. But what is different is the lightness of spirit and sweetness of love contained in the new covenant of Christ. This is brought about through an alchemical transformation with lighter herbal essences.

Compassion was revealed as a blend of aromas that harmonize love and intelligence. This fusion evokes the higher consciousness of compassion. There are wild roses in this that grow on the hills of Arabia and are hand picked by the maidens who live there. Then they are blended with other essences that gently stimulate the brain and bring it into harmony with the heart.

Innocence is the sweet fragrance of the soul, forever young and reborn eternally in the presence of the Holy Spirit. It is a complex blend with Lotus flower as one of its ingredients. Lotus has long been regarded in Eastern traditions as the flower that blossoms through the touch of God.

Forgiveness is a pure and uplifting fragrance that has Lilly of the Valley for one of its ingredients. Its regal simplicity reminds us that God is our true authority and all else is fleeting experience. True forgiveness does not deny the error, but learns from it, and transcends to a higher life of greater goodness.

Peace is as rare and exquisite as the state of being it invokes. Indescribably gentle, it elicits a response from the higher states of relaxed consciousness, and releases the tensions of chaotic overload, sometimes encountered in the physical world of ordinary endeavor and thought. Peace is not when you successfully bring order to the world, but when you bring serenity to yourself.

Abundance invokes a spicy and rich assurance of infinite supply. Its foundation is gratitude. Far beyond the prosperity of material acquisition, abundance encompasses all the wealth of creation and the human experience. The unconditional state of abundance expands through sharing and caring.

Joy brings the scent of flowering life in springtime. Joy is the soul's celebration of being the love that it is—a blessing to the world, yet not of the world. Knowing this brings joy. Unlike happiness, joy is not bound to pleasure and other needs for positive reward. Joy is the soul's exhalation regardless of circumstances.

Wisdom develops when all of these states of unconditional being are focused into complete acceptance and knowing. In Greek, the word for wisdom is Sophia. Many scriptures refer to wisdom as "precious," "sacred," and "feminine." Solomon expressed this principle beautifully in the Book of Proverbs (Ch. 8). This not to imply that wisdom is not a prized virtue among men. It does suggest that wisdom comes when we strive for completeness and balance in all things.

Other Sacred Blends for Inspiration and Guidance:

Om is a fragrance that takes us into a state of reverence and preparedness to receive sacred revelations or healing. It opens the Sacred Heart and all the other sacred centers where body, mind, and spirit connect. It is appropriate to use this before prayer or meditation, or in any communion with the Divine. It can be used in combination with any of the other oils.

Holy Ground is a serene but vibrant fragrance reminiscent of high mountain air with a hint of wild flowers. It was created to help you leave the world below as you ascend into higher states of prayer and meditation.

Love is a fragrance that whispers "you are loved" without uttering a word! With the Sacred Oil "Love" you can literally radiate the presence of love. It will be recognized on a subtle level by everyone...even those who are afraid to believe or trust in love. Although it has some floral top notes of rose and jasmine, it is not exclusively feminine.